Ted Holloway

THE 4-MINUTE WORKOUT

Challenging Mindsets to get You up and Moving

ACKNOWLEDGEMENTS

First of all, I want to give thanks to my Heavenly Father who strengthens and sustains me each and everyday. It isn't easy being self-employed, but through Him I can achieve anything. Secondly, my wife who lets me be the eagle that can fly as high as I like. Furthermore, to my consultant, Tamika Hall, who convinced me to put my many ideas on paper. I especially want to thank Shannon Crist, Heather Miciche, Amanda Newell and Kelly Byrd who encouraged me and walked through the doors with me when I decided to pursue my dream of owning my own fitness and personal training studio. Hey Pat McMullen! Thanks for opening your doors to me and my Warrior Dash family along with my loyal and dedicated middle and high school athletes.

TABLE OF CONTENTS

INTRODUCTION

When I think about the blessings I've had to experience so many different things that have made me who I am today, I am thankful to have experienced things such as: owning two gyms, being a US Marine and Army Veteran, competing in bodybuilding shows, training people for competitions, coaching high school and college track and field, college football, head strength and conditioning coach, and in 2013 owning a gym again. Out of these experiences the Holloway Formula was created. I have been blessed to be very successful in every experience I have had from coaching state champions to producing NFL players, and even more gratifying helping people meet their fitness goals.

I hope this book will encourage many people to understand the importance of getting fit. I hope to inspire Pastor's to take a look at my program so that they can encourage their members to start the change, convince their members to strengthen spirit, mind, body and soul with the 4-minute workout.

Let me be clear! This book and workout plan is about helping people make those small changes that's doable and measurable. It's starting a change. It's about learning how to commit, to not make excuses about why they won't workout or learn to eat healthy.

With so many experiences, I used the Holloway Formula to develop workouts for the everyday fitness enthusiasts to world-class athletes. The Holloway Formula truly is a multi-dimensional workout plan. I'm often asked how do I get rid of this body fat? I'm often told, "I don't have time to workout," or "I don't want to spend hours in the gym."

I tell them, "Heck! I don't want to spend hours in the gym either whether training myself or other people!" There are some good programs out there that I personally think are awesome and less than an hour. A few great celebrity trainers have recently went as far as reducing programs to ten minutes and people still say they don't have time.

How did the 4-Minute Workout come about? Well, I went a step further. After spending many hours in the gym I designed short workouts that some of my fittest clients felt were taxing and the 4-minute workout. Listen, my friends, this is it! None of us trainers can do any better than this. I know it works because I have had clients who couldn't do one round in four minutes. However, as they have become more fit and followed the eating plan, the change in body composition happened. It also prepared them to slowly increase their ability to do more and eventually complete the next tier workouts as well as helped increased their metabolisms. This was evident based off of their continued weight loss.

I'm not telling you that the 4, 7, 12, 16 and 20 minute workouts aren't challenging, but what I am telling you is **the four minute time limit allows you to start somewhere that you can do it twice per day whether that is** by yourself in the morning and with the family in the afternoon. It allows time for the family to do something healthy together as well as learn to eat healthy after such a powerful and challenging workout. My hope is that once they see that they are getting stronger and more fit they will want to continue challenging themselves not only when completing their workouts but also making better food choices.

The workouts in this book are designed for the post-partum mom, for the busy person, for the person who swears they just don't have time to workout, people who do not like or have time for gyms, and finally for those people that find it very difficult to get through some of the new workouts created by celebrity fitness trainers. I'm trying to bridge the gap by creating workouts that are quick and will hopefully lead people down the road to challenge themselves to more advanced and longer workouts. The 4-Minute workout is just the beginning to your fitness journey. I will be offering several workout programs: The 4-Minute Mommy workout, The 4-Minute Family workout, and The 4-Minute Healthy Beginnings workout.

The purpose of my book is not to overload you with all these technical terms used in exercise science and by all these so called fitness experts. If that's what you want you can contact me by email or Facebook me and schedule a time with me and I'll be glad to help educate you. I learned from in my opinion from one of the best trainers in the country, Jeff "Maddog" Madden that people don't want to be bogged down with technical science jargon they want to know, "Can you help me get to my goals? Can you make me be fit? Can you help me become the best athlete I can be or the best in the world?"

So I want to accomplish two things in this book. First, just get people moving. Second, is to get people to change the way they are thinking about working out and being healthy. The goal is to start with small changes. Forgive me but you cannot convince me that you can't find four minutes per day for five days per week. The beauty of the program is you could actually repeat it day and night until you get to tier 3 of which we will talk more about when we come to the workout programs.

This book isn't meant to compete or bash other fitness expert's philosophy. The development of this program is from my many hours and years spent in the gym with my clients and much feedback from the people that took my classes as well as the many people I have been blessed to help. Therefore this is my own philosophy and opinion. I was encouraged to develop such a program from much listening and from feedback from clients to people who really wanted to train with me but was either to busy, unmotivated or to intimidated being in a gym setting. So guess what everyone? I listened.

One thing most trainers fail to tell people is the start to a healthy lifestyle is small subtle changes and then getting you moving. Keep in mind you really must want this. You really must want to live. You really have to be sick and tired of being sick and tired. Some things we *can* control. I beg you please do not wait until your doctor tells you that you now have high blood pressure, borderline diabetes, high cholesterol or anything else. The reason is that once they inform you of this condition you can rest assure they are going to put you on medications. Don't depend on these medications they will lead to something else. Don't be content taking unnecessary medications when you can do the necessary things to at least show your doctor that you are taking the proper steps to be a healthier you. You never know they just might either lower the dosage or take you off all together. No claims or promises here. I just know most good doctors will tell you to do exactly what I'm telling you: make changes to your EATING and MOVE!

BODYWEIGHT EXERCISES

The following is list of bodyweight exercises I personally feel will get you the best results for burning fat and will help amp up your metabolism along with following clean eating and drinking close to a gallon of water per day. In my Appendix I will give you an example of how I ate when I was competing and how I eat now for weight loss and overall wellness. Again this is a list of bodyweight exercises I personally use in my own gym:

- Mountain Climbers
- Jump roping and Jump modifications
- Burpee variations and modifications
- Squat Jumps
- Lunge Jumps
- Box Jumps if available
- Walk-outs and the many combinations that go with this movement
- (Push-ups, planks, lunges, Spiderman step, Mt. Climber variations)
- Shuttles
- Shuffle
- Wood Chops

- Dumbbell movements and combinations
- Squat variations (air, goblet, dumbbell)
- Push-ups and modifications and push-up progressions

There are also boxing workouts that are amazing providing you have the equipment however you can improvise that as well. You will see that at the end of the workout programs. I totally believe in bodyweight exercises from my days as a Marine. If budget permits I would like for you to invest in:

- Jump rope
- Yoga Mat
- Women: 5,10 and 15 lbs. dumbbells
- Men: 15, 20 and 25lb dumbbells

Parents, this is a great program for your children who play sports but don't like to go to the gym once the season is over. This program will be great for them to stay in shape especially if they can make it to Tier 5 between seasons. Some kids play a sport and when it is over they sit around and play video games until the next season. Parents, I REPEAT, don't let your kid sit around and do nothing! If for nothing else you can help possibly lower their chances of getting injured. As a coach there is nothing more satisfying than seeing an athlete show up in great shape. On the flip side there is nothing more disturbing then to see a kid come in totally out of shape

Burpee Variations

Next are all the many Burpee variations. I'm sure there are more; it boils down to imagination, safety and creativeness of the trainer:

- Half Burpee (keep in mind that you find that the same exercises used by different trainers may have different names. This movement is sometimes referred to as the bend and thrust or pike Burpee depending if the emphasis is on abs or conditioning or both)
- Burpee push-up
- Burpee combined with dumbbell shoulder press
- The Double Burpee is an advance movement and requires a lot of strength and endurance
- Triple Burpee combined with walkout to 3 push-ups then back up
- Half Burpee push-up
- 2-minute Burpee challenge (30 correct position Burpees meaning Burpee to perfect push-up position back up with jump
- 2-minute Burpee push-up (again perfect push-up position BACK STRAIGHT)
- Burpee Pyramid 10,9,8...1

Note: all of the advance movements should not be attempted until you perfect the basics such as safety, correct body position and posture.

For video demonstrations of all exercises visit my website. There is also a complete workout of one of my 4-Minute workouts so you can see how it should be completed. I will post one of an individual and one with a group so you can see how intense yet fun it can be as well as help you organize your group or even your family.

WARM-UP

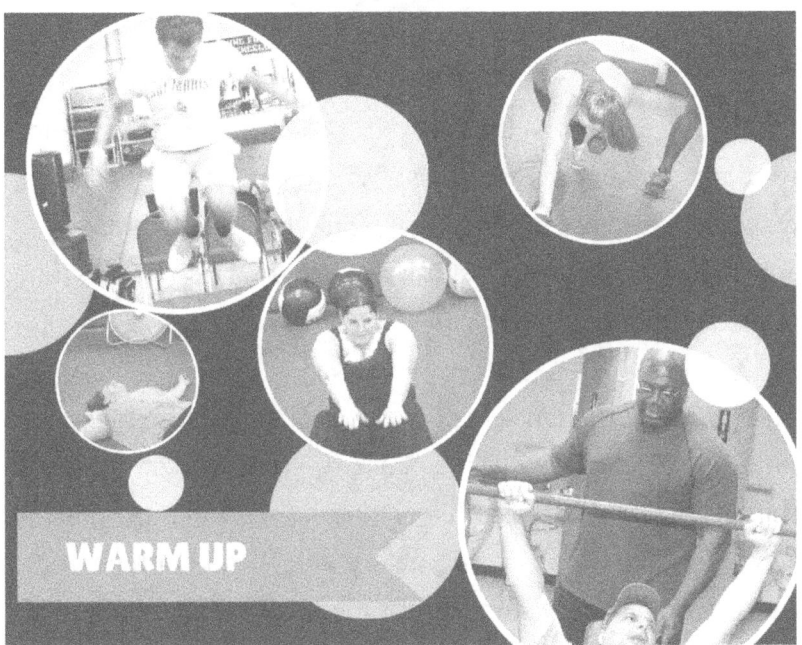

Some trainers and critics are going to ask, "Where is the warm up?" First, I will tell them if they ever do this workout they will see after one or two intense rounds of this you are warmed up. No need to fret. I like to use my TR combination warm up it's similar to the TR workout yet different.

The warm up is:

- 20 reach and toe touches
- 20 single count jumping jacks
- 30 seconds of running in place.

This should take about two minutes. Once completed you will start the 4-Minute Workout.

Once you get through the six-week program you will start to see the method of my madness. When you get to Tier Two it will all make sense to you. You won't have to explain a thing. If one is curious just ask them to do the workout with you.

This TR combination set is a workout unto itself because you can do so much with it. At my gym we do pyramid challenges for time with this combo set. I don't recommend attempting challenges until you are able to do ten reps of the entire series without stopping for more then 30 seconds. This is the sequence of movements in the TR combination set:

- Always start with 10 Jumping Jacks (beginners always start with single count JJs meaning 1,2,3,.. 10. As you get more advanced begin to use two count cadence or double the total amount for example; 10 JJs will actually be 20)
- Walk-out then from the push-up position twist to left and right planks for about one second each side
- Push-up,
- Spiderman step,

- Walk back up,
- Lunge with the left leg and back repeat with right leg,
- 1 dumbbell thruster, then 10 JJs

That whole sequence is one rep.

To pyramid this you would on the second set do 2 of everything then 3,4,5 and so on depending on the prescribed workout of the day. This is very advanced so work your way through the single sequence for a set of 10 reps. Remember the entire combo is one rep.

You can also pyramid the planks. For example; 1:00, :50, :40, :30, :20, :10 each side with a 30 second break between transitions.

4-MINUTE EXERCISES PLANS

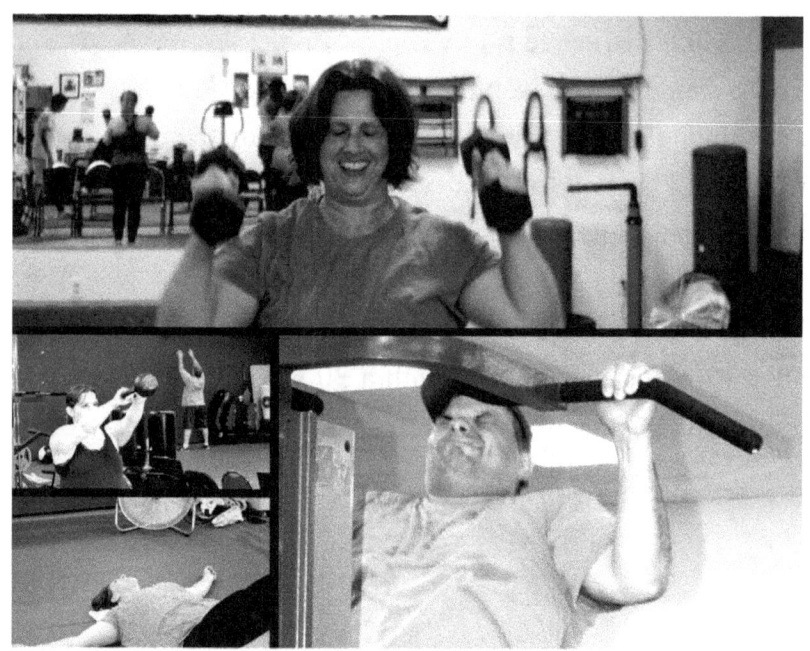

LET'S GO!

The beauty of my short workouts is they are all measurable in that each workout and each week you will see improvements both from a fitness and weight loss standpoint as long as you follow the program consistently along with the eating clean. Keep in mind the purpose is to get you moving and making those subtle changes with the hopes that they will gradually become habit then a lifestyle. The workouts can be for time or just to challenge yourself for completion.

It's very important to keep a journal on your progressions. A journal has been provided after each week's exercise. I also recommend using MYFITNESS PAL to record everything you eat each day. It's an invaluable tool and it's a free app to download.

Most of the workouts require bodyweight only, however, there are instances where minimal equipment is required. The investment will be well worth it. Everything from supplements to equipment will add value to your life. Again think of it all as an investment to prolong your life. Once you complete the six-week training program the next week try completing three rounds in all the 4-Minute Workouts from week one. So lets get ready for weeks 1-6 (4 MINUTES LETS GO)!

WEEK ONE

In four minutes try to complete the entire block as many times as possible.

DAY	EXERCISES	HOW DID YOU DO?
Monday **ROCK'S 7s**	• Jumping Jacks 2 count or 14 total • Push-ups • Knee outside • Mt. Climbers 2 count or 14 total • Burpees • 70 jump rope singles with rope or modified version without rope	
Tuesday **TED'S 10s**	• 10 Mt. Climbers 2 count or 20 total • Plank alternating arm extensions from push-up position (one on each side for total of 20.) • 10 Walkouts • 10 Squat jumps • 10 step lunge walk each leg	
Wednesday: 2-Minute Burpee challenge 30 Burpees in 2 minutes keep going until you can do 30 Burpees in 2 minutes.		

THE 4-MINUTE WORKOUT

DAY	EXERCISES	HOW DID YOU DO?
Thursday 33 ON Thursday	• 33 Jumping Jacks • 33 sit-ups • 33 jump rope singles • 3 push-ups • 3 Mt. climbers • 3 plank alternating arm extensions • 3T-Twist • 3 outside Mt. Climbers	
Friday Fun Friday	20 seconds of work; 10 seconds rest (Tabatas) • Plank. Attempt to do 8 rounds • End with 50 two count Jumping Jacks or total of 100	
Saturday	In the morning try the 2-Minute Burpee challenge again. Record in your journal your progress.	

Starting Weight: _____

Measurements:

Waist: _____ Hips: _____

Don't get caught up in checking your weight everyday because it fluctuates.

WEEK TWO

DAY	EXERCISES	HOW DID YOU DO?
Monday **"MOANING MONDAY"**	• 5 Squat Jumps • 5 walkout push-ups • 5 Bends and Thrust • 5 Pyramid sit-up/leg lift combo • 50 Jump rope singles	
Tuesday **TED'S 10s**	• Run in place for 30 seconds rest 15 seconds • Plank all 3 sides for 30seconds no rest. Transition right into left side • Air Squat for 30 seconds with 15 second rest • Run in place 30 seconds rest 15 seconds. This may go a bit over 4 minutes.	
Wednesday: 2 minute Burpee challenge 30 Burpees in 2 minutes keep going until you can do 30 Burpees in 2 minutes.		

YOU CAN DO IT! YOU ARE HALFWAY THERE

Are you getting any faster and fit? Have you made some changes? Did you weigh in? You should start to feel changes happening. You should be looking to make some new changes. Your cheat day is coming. Two more

days until Saturday.		
DAY	**EXERCISES**	**HOW DID YOU DO?**
Thursday Thirsty Thursday	:20/:10 rest Squats-Jumping Jacks-Push-ups-Burpees repeat sequence immediately. The goal here is to be able to do each one of these for 8 rounds attempting to tie or beat your highest number. This is a true Tabata workout.	
Friday 10x10 Friday	Walkouts, Bends and Thrust, Squat Jumps, Thrusters (5,8,10lb dumbbells)	

SATURDAY- CHEAT DAY

It's your cheat day! Some trainers and so-called experts may disagree with this. It's a very controversial top. That's their opinion. I'm a former bodybuilder who used my cheat day to keep my sanity. I didn't have any problems getting right back on track. Although I have trained many clients who are mentally tough with a lot of will power. However, I will caution you. If you are one of these all or nothing people then you have to be completely honest with yourself about having a cheat day or cheat meal. I don't want my clients beating themselves up for having a cheat meal or even a cheat day. I want them to communicate with me so I can get them back on track immediately. It's important that you are honest with yourself and your trainer. Should you find yourself falling you can contact me via email or Facebook, which I will give that information at the end of this book.

All good trainers want feedback and honesty on your part so that they can help you or in this case I can help you. Now don't get me wrong, some of you may be strong enough not to warrant a cheat day or may feel like you haven't worked hard enough during your first two weeks of training. Again be honest with yourself. Ask yourself could I have given it more? Could I have completed another four minute set or at least half? Am I really trying to eat clean and often? Is my water intake up?

Enjoy your cheat day, because Week Three is just two days away ☺

WEEK THREE

DAY	EXERCISES	HOW DID YOU DO?
Monday 4X4	4 rounds of each 20 seconds work/10 seconds rest • Run in place • Dumbbell or Kettlebell swings • Sumo Deadlifts • Plank alternating arm extensions	
Tuesday	• :30 Jump Rope or Jumping Jacks • Rest :15 • :30 Push-ups • :15 rest Total of 5 minutes includes rest	
Wednesday: 2-Minute Burpee Challenge 30 Burpees in 2 minutes keep going until you can do 30 Burpees in 2 minutes. Are you any closer to getting 30 Burpees in 2 minutes? (Remember each Burpee must be done correctly meaning you must go to a perfect push-up position each rep) record in your journal how many you completed		

DAY	EXERCISES	HOW DID YOU DO?
Thursday	• Set timer for 5 minutes do as many sets of these as you can in 5 minutes • 7 Squats • 7 walkouts • 7 Half Burpees • 7 Mt. Climbers • 70 Jump rope singles • Record how many rounds you completed	
Friday Fun Friday	8 Pyramid up Squat-Curl-press Set your timer for 4 minutes record where you stopped	
Saturday	CHEAT MEAL- Choose just ONE meal that you will cheat on	

WEEK 4

Let's repeat some workouts from week one to see where you stand from your journal recordings

DAY	EXERCISES	Record
Monday 4X4	• 5 walkout push-ups • 5 sit-ups • 5 plank alternating arm extensions • 25 JJs • 5 Squats	
Tuesday **Ted's Giant** **Set Combo**	10 single count JJs-walkout-T-twist L/R-push-up-Spiderman step L/R-walk back up- left leg lunge then right leg lunge-Thruster-10 single count JJs this is one set (This will be a pyramid workout as well. It can be descending or ascending)	
Wednesday: Jump rope Tabata try to get 38-40 touches per: 20 seconds. Once you gain the skill you will find this very challenging.		
Thursday	100- 2 Count JJs or 200- 3x12 half Burpees	
Friday	3x: 30 3 side planks complete sequence 2 more times if possible finish with 50 Jumping Jacks	
Saturday	Do your Burpee challenge again.	

WEEK 5

DAY	EXERCISES	Record
Monday 4X4	Estimate about 10ft of space shuffle left do Burpee shuffle right do Burpee for :30 then rest :30, next high knee for :30 then rest :30, next do :30 of knee outside Mountain Climbers followed by :30 of rest, next :30 of plank alternating arm extensions followed by :30 of rest (*You can modify each of these exercises as well as work your way up to the :30)	
Tuesday **3 Rounds**	• 6 Squat jumps • 6 back step lunges each leg • 6 half-Burpees • 6 push-up combined with alternating arm extensions • 60 jump rope singles	
Wednesday **10x10**	• Jumping Jacks • Air Squats • Forward step lunge then back step lunge • Double Burpee Do as many rounds as possible in 4 minutes	
Thursday: Tabata :20 with :10 rest for 8 rounds Push-ups, walk outs, jump lunges, squat jumps, jumping jacks, high knees, sit-ups, plank alternating arm extensions		

THE 4-MINUTE WORKOUT

Friday	• 50 Jump rope singles • 50 sit-ups • 50 jump rope singles • 10 push-ups • 10 knees outside elbow mountain climbers • 10 half Burpees • 50 Jump rope singles	
Saturday	CHEAT MEAL- Remember to pick just ONE meal	

WEEK 6

We are in week six and if you have been seriously and consistently following the program you are now highly skilled in doing the movements and should be pretty strong by now. The beauty of this type of training is that you see yourself get stronger and fit. You may even start to feel as though you could do another round. You can also repeat this workout in the afternoon with your family. Just remind them it's only 4 minutes. So let's finish week six.

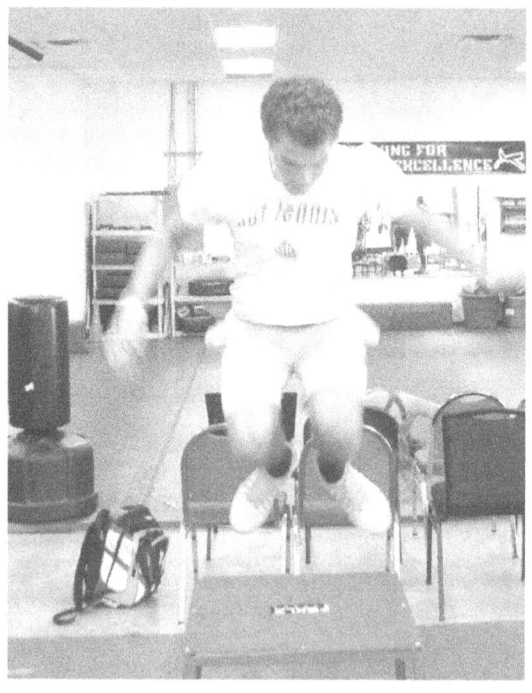

THE 4-MINUTE WORKOUT

DAY	EXERCISES	Record
Monday	• 7 15ft shuttles • 7 cross body mountain climbers • 7 spinal rolls • 7 side hops over and back is one rep (note use a pencil or ruler to jump over) • :30 of high knees take a :30 rest immediately begin round two.	
Tuesday	This is very challenging, but it's week 6 you can handle it. Try this Non-stop • 15 Burpees • 15 Mt. Climbers count each side • 15 squat-curl-press • 15 boxing 1/2s as fast as you can should equal 30 punches total • 15 lunges each leg 15 Jumping Jacks	
Wednesday	Burpee challenge: 30 Burpees in 2 minutes	
Thursday	• 5 prison squats • 5 shuttles • 5 push-ups • 5 squats • 5 half -Burpee with plank alternating arm extensions • 50 Jumping Jacks	

Friday	Tabatas :20/:10 rest Push-up followed by Plank repeat for a total of 8 rounds (note: alternate the two exercises)	
Saturday	Final Burpee challenge: 30 Burpees in 2 minutes. You should be close now.	

YOU MADE IT!

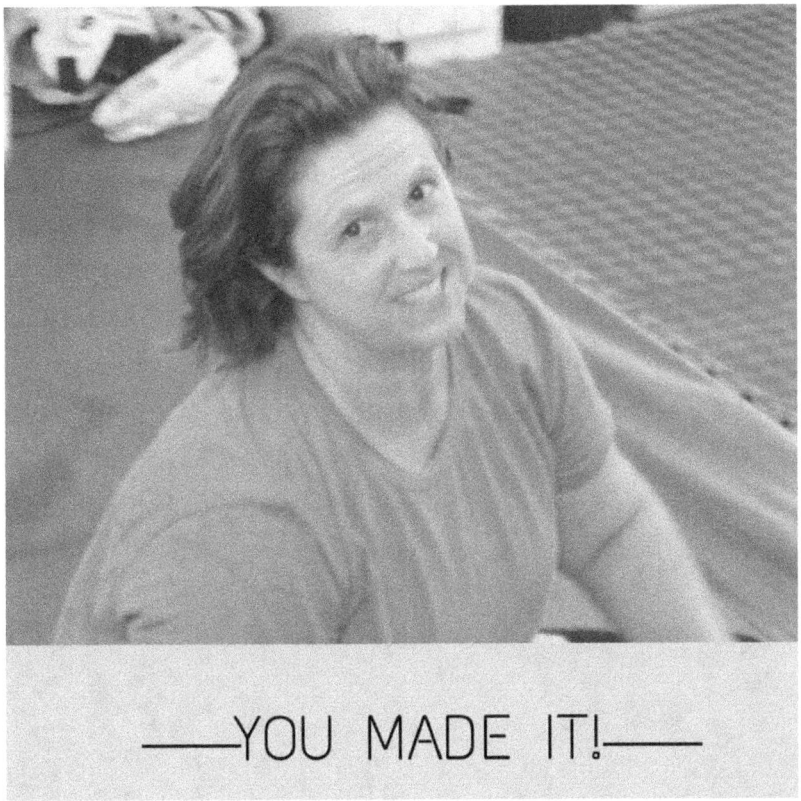

——YOU MADE IT!——

Now that you have completed this six-week program go back over your journal and see where you struggled. Try to repeat those workouts where you didn't get at least 2 1/2-3 rounds. Ideally, I would like to see you complete at least 2 complete rounds of every four-minute AMRAP (as many rounds as possible) before moving on to Tier 2, which will be a seven-minute AMRAP. Being a Marine we use many acronyms.

The AMRAP is a popular acronym used by the Crossfit community and its founder is Dr. Glassman.

I cannot emphasis enough that this program is designed to get you moving as well as start to be consistent with your daily and weekly workouts. Think of it this way; your workouts will challenge you in the same way life will. When it gets hard are you going to quit? When you don't feel like it are you still going to do it? No different than when you are tired and have to go to work. You still go right? It's those days when you don't feel like it you sometimes have your best workouts. It also makes you feel like you have accomplished something. Kind of a gratifying feeling that only you can appreciate.

APPENDIX: MEAL PLAN & PORTION CONTROL

My own meal plan that I personally used to get me ripped for my bodybuilding competitions and how I eat now. Should you decide to follow this sample be sure to check with your doctor as I am a firm believer in supplementation you or your doctor may not be. Again this is how I personally eat and I just want to share with you what a days meal plan looks like as a competitor and for health and wellness. One thing to remember is our food isn't what it used to be. Our palates are so messed up because of genetically engineered food and its high sugar content. When we attempt to eat clean we are programmed to believe that it tastes awful and in many cases makes you feel like you are depriving yourself of something. Eating healthy shouldn't make you feel that way. Learning how to be creative in the kitchen will go a long way in helping you and your family enjoy eating healthy.

If you are serious about your weight loss and wellness please invest in a FOOD SCALE. I cannot stress enough, weigh your food and know your portions. Your portions may vary depending on your activity levels.

Evaluate this meal plan carefully tell me what you noticed

COMPETITION MEAL PLAN

A typical Monday for competition:

7:15am 40 minutes of cardio

Breakfast: 8am

- My supplements
- Bowl of oatmeal
- Large fruit
- 8 egg whites 2 whole eggs
- 20ozs of water (some times a cup of black coffee or green tea)

10:30am- small can of tuna and fruit

Lunch-12:45

- Chicken breast
- Vegetable or salad
- Yam or Sweet potato
- 20oz bottle of water
- Supplements

Nap 1:45-2:30

2:45pm Late afternoon snack

- Hand full of Almonds or Walnuts or Protein Shake (sometimes both)

4:30pm Pre-Workout supplement

5:00pm cardio
5:30pm weight training
20oz cup of water most times more
6:30pm small fruit

Dinner 7:00pm
- Haddock
- Asparagus
- Yam or brown rice

(Sometimes I may have an extra protein shake mixed with water only depending on the intensity of my workout)

Snack 9:00pm air popcorn or 1 cup of sherbert 20oz cup of water

Sleep 10:15pm

HEALTH/WELLNESS AND WEIGHT LOSS

Monday

Breakfast: 8:00am

- Supplements
- Bowl of oatmeal or 3 hard boiled eggs (sometimes a chicken breast)
- Medium size piece of fruit
- Coffee or green tea
- 20ozs or more of water

10:30am a high quality snack bar

20ozs of water

11:00am pre-workout supplements

11:30am workout

20ozs of water or more

12:30pm Lunch

- Large salad with some sort of protein: turkey breast, chicken, steak, or tuna (NO LUNCH MEAT it is full of salt, fat, and harmful preservatives). dressing balsamic vinegar, medium fruit, Ice tea

3:00pm
- High protein meal bar
- 20ozs of water

4:30pm pre-workout supplement
5:00pm
Occasionally I have to workout at this time

6:00pm medium fruit after workout
20ozs of water

7:00pm Dinner
- Lean 9oz steak
- Jasmine rice or brown rice
- Broccoli, asparagus, collar greens, kale, green beans
Semi-sweet tea (Note: not suggesting alcohol but if I'm within my calories I will have red or white wine depending on the meat I'm eating)

Again, I just gave you an example of how my wife and I may eat on a daily basis. If you are one of these people who have to have wine with your meals or late night when reading a book it is important that you workout and stay within your portions so there is room for a glass or two of wine. If you are a heavy drinker and you are trying to stop, then it wouldn't be wise to have wine at all at.

Please don't make excuses about your kids. My kids eat whatever my wife and I eat. We allow them to be kids, but we carefully monitor how much junk they are allowed. My youngest is very cunning when it comes to sweets so we have to really keep an eye on her when she is allowed to have those treats.

You don't have to be miserable when eating clean. You can be very creative as well as use a variety of tasty seasonings when cooking and that is why my kids enjoy eating the way we eat. I have several resources to share with you if you need advice on clean eating recipes, or how to conduct your own eat clean workshops. Now as I told you earlier I'm very big on supplementation. I don't care what other trainers say or believe this is just what I believe. I've spent years researching the best supplement companies and I firmly believe in the one I and all my clients use. If you are interested in more information on what I use email or Facebook message me and I will be glad to give you more information. I believe in bridging the gap to get the nutrients I cannot get from our food. Please don't misunderstand what

I'm saying. YOU NEED FOOD. SUPPLEMENTS OR SHAKES DON'T REPLACE FOOD. SHAKES ARE GREAT AND CONVENIENT FOR THE BUSY PERSON, BUT YOU NEED FOOD, GOOD FOOD.

I want everyone to understand that as a trainer I want to help people. I also understand you have to meet people where they are. That's why I created programs for people who are busy and do not have a lot of time but really want to workout. With the 4-Minute Workout there is little room for excuses. There are some people who flat out won't workout and have no problem living off prescribed medications that in many cases can be avoided with good eating and exercise. I just want to get people moving so this is why I'm really pushing the 4-Minute Workout. As I told you in the beginning of this book, I get a lot of feedback from people that say they buy all these workout programs from celebrity fitness trainers – which in my opinion are great, but they say I can't get through them so they get down on themselves and quit. At that point the products becomes a waste of money and ends up on the shelf collecting dust.

The 4-Minute Workout won't cost you an arm and a leg. It is very affordable and you get lots of support. Once you purchase my eBook and read through it you can go to my website and see all the exercise demonstrations. Keep in mind no one owns any exercise movements. So you will see some of the same exercises everywhere however like most good trainers I used my imagination to get very creative in the advance movements which I believe will greatly enhance your strength, skill, coordination and fitness levels. More importantly burn mounds of fat. My program will help you reach your goals if you are consistent and honest with yourself on how much you put into it. So whether you decide to stick with my program or any other they will have properly prepared you to take on such challenging and intense workouts.

I hope you enjoy the workouts and remember they can be done two more times per day. Do them with your family. Do with your friends and church group. Just get moving and eating clean my friends and become a healthier you. Start small and gradually increase to the next 4 Tiers. So let's have fun and spread the word. Lets get people moving and healthy.

ABOUT THE AUTHOR

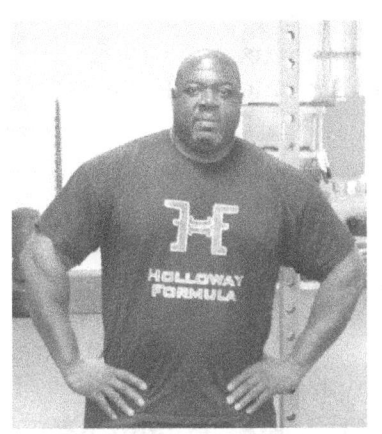 **TED HOLLOWAY, an** award winning fitness trainer, received his Bachelor of Specialized Studies with Emphasis on Physical Education from Ohio University. He went on to complete a Master's Degree in Organizational Management from Ashford University

He is a certified Sports Performance Level I Coach through USA Weight Lifting and Crossfit Level I. He has obtained the highest certification in Sports Conditioning (MSS, Master Of Sports Science).

Coach Holloway teaches a philosophy known as "Explosive Power," which was taught to him by his mentor, Jeff "Mad Dog" Madden, longtime Strength and Conditioning Director at the University of Texas. He is a strong believer in mental toughness training, which he personally benefited from during his service with the U.S. Marine Corps. Coach Holloway was also a Division 1 football and track and field coach. In his time there, he has coached several world-class athletes including several students who went on to the NFL. He has coached numerous state champions and top six finishers in track and field.

Coach Holloway has received several awards including:

- What's Up Eastern Shore Magazine 2014 & 2013 Best Personal Trainer at a Private Studio

- What's Up Eastern Shore Magazine 2014 & 2013 Best Children's Fitness Program

- 2013 Shore Update Newspaper Best Freelance Trainer

Over the years, Coach Holloway has been hired by and taught various types of athletes, which is why he no longer refers to himself as strength and conditioning coach, but a developmental coach. Coach Rock won't just improve your body, but your mind and emotions as well. He is certified in Anger Management and Conflict Resolution and has spent a lot of time working with many athletes and teens in dealing with their anger issues. Coach Holloway states, "Bring me Heart and Desire and I will make you 100% better."

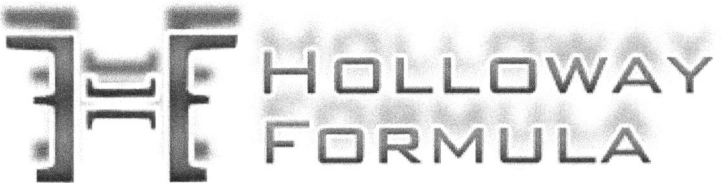

STAY CONNECTED!

For video demonstrations:
www.hollowayformula.com

Email:
ted@HollowayFormula.com

Twitter
www.twitter.com / hollowayformula

Facebook
www.facebook.com / hollowayformula

NOTES

NOTES

NOTES

www.ingramcontent.com/pod-product-compliance
Lightning Source LLC
Chambersburg PA
CBHW070230290526
45789CB00004B/1556

* 9 7 8 1 5 0 0 1 3 8 7 3 8 *